ATKINS DIET

Ultimate Guide To The Atkins Diet For Beginners Everything
You Need To Know About The Atkins Diet

(Atkins Diet Recipes For Beginners)

Toby Mcdaniel

TABLE OF CONTENTS

Low-Carb Lasagna

Ingredients

- 2 tsp leaf Oregano

- 2 large Fresh fresh fresh eggs

- 2 tsp leaf Basil

- 1/5 tsp leaf Dried Thyme Leaves

- 1/5 cup Tap Water

- 1/10 tsp Black Pepper

- 5 cup Large or Small Curd Creamed Cottage Cheese

- 2   cup shredded Mozzarella Cheese 1/25 cup 100% Stone Ground Whole Wheat Pastry Flour

- 2 medium Zucchinis

- 2 lb. Ground Beef

- 1/5 cup chopped Fresh onion s

- 2 1/5 cup chopped or sliced Red Tomatoes

- 2 can Tomato Paste

- 2 tsp Garlic

Directions

1. Cook zucchini until tender, drain and set aside.

2. Fry meat and fresh onion s until meat is brown and fresh onion s are tender; drain fat.

3. Add next 8 ingredients and bring to a boil.
4. Reduce heat; simmer, uncovered 10 minutes or until reduced to 2 cups.
5. In a small bowl slightly beat fresh fresh fresh eggs .
6. Add cottage cheese, half of shredded cheese and flour.

7. In a 2 2 -qt. baking/roasting pan arrange half of the meat mixture.
8. Top with half of the zucchini and all the cottage cheese mixture.
9. Top with remaining meat and zucchini.
10. Bake uncovered at 4 8 6 °F for 45 minutes.
11. Sprinkle with remaining cheese and bake 10 minutes longer.

12.   Let stand for 10 minutes before serving.

Fresh Berry Tarts With Cream

Ingredients

- 1/5 cup Heavy Cream
- 2 cup Red Raspberries
- 2 tbsps. Sucralose Based Sweetener
- 3 cup, slivered Almonds
- 2 cup Fresh Blueberries

Directions

1. Heat broiler.
2. Chop almonds and divide among 4 small ramekins.
3. Sprinkle 2 tablespoon sugar substitute over the almonds.
4. Place ramekins on a cookie sheet and broil until the tops of the nuts

are golden and the sugar substitute has melted.

5. Remove and cool until at room temperature.
6. Whip the heavy cream and remaining tablespoon of sugar substitute until doubled in volume.
7. Place one-quarter of blueberries and one-quarter of raspberries in each ramekin and top with a dollop of whipped cream.
8. Serve immediately.

Farmers Breakfast Soup

Ingredients

- 3 cup High Protein TVP
- 2 cup chopped Celery
- 2 cup chopped Carrots
- 4 cups Chicken Broth, Bouillon or Consomme
- 1/5 tsp Black Pepper
- 2 cup chopped Fresh onion s
- 2 medium slice Bacon
- 8 oz. Turkey Sausage
- 4 oz. Ground Beef

Directions

1. In a large non-stick skillet, over medium heat, cook the bacon until it begins to brown.

2. Add the sausage and beef to brown, breaking up the meat into small bits with a spatula or spoon.
3. Stir in the TVP and vegetables.
4. Cook 6 minutes until vegetables begin to soften.
5. Add remaining ingredients and simmer for 25 minutes, skimming off excess fat from the surface of the liquid.
6. Season with salt and pepper to taste.

Mini Chocolate Chip Muffins

Ingredients

- 2 tbsps. Unsalted Butter Stick
- 2 tbsps. Heavy Cream
- 2 fl oz. Tap Water
- 2 tsps. Vanilla Extract
- 4 oz. Sugar Free Chocolate Chips
- 2 cup Whole Grain Soy Flour
- 2 tsp Baking Powder
- 2 cup Sucralose Based Sweetener
- 1/5 tsp Salt
- 2 cup Sour Cream

Directions

1. Heat oven to 4 6 0°F.
2. Grease two 12-compartment mini muffin pans.

3. In a bowl, combine soy flour, baking powder, sugar substitute, and salt.
4. In another bowl, whisk sour cream, butter, heavy cream, water and vanilla to combine.
5. Add the sour cream mixture to the soy mixture.
6. Stir until well combined.
7. Fold in chocolate chips.
8. Divide batter in pan compartments, using about 2 rounded tablespoon per muffin.
9. Bake 16 -25 minutes, or until lightly browned on top and toothpick inserted in center comes out clean.
10. Cool muffins in pans for 2 minutes, then turn out onto wire racks to cool completely.

Power "Oatmeal"

Ingredients

- 1/5 tsp Cinnamon
- 2 cup Large or Small Curd Creamed Cottage Cheese
- 2 oz. Vanilla Whey Protein
- 4 oz. Dry Textured Vegetable Protein
- 2 14 oz. can Coconut Cream
- 2 cup Tap Water

Directions

1. Note: You can find textured vegetable proteinin any natural foods store or in some well-stocked supermarkets.
2. In this recipe its texture suggests oatmeal.

3. Combine the textured vegetable protein, coconut milk, water, cinnamon, protein powder and cottage cheese in a large saucepan with a heavy bottom.
4. Cook, over low heat, for 25 minutes, or until mixture has thickened and is tender.
5. Serve with a little cream and sugar substitute, if desired.

Blueberry-Turkey Burgers

Ingredients

- 2 2 tsps. Cumin
- 2 tsp Salt
- 2 tsp Black Pepper
- 2 cup chopped Red Sweet Pepper
- 5 cup crumbled Feta Cheese
- 5 cup Blueberries
- 2 1/5 lbs. Ground Turkey
- 2 tbsp. Light Olive Oil
- 4 tbsps. Peppermint
- 2 2 tsps. Fennel Seed

Directions

1. Ground turkey can be dry, adding additional olive oil is optional but the

bell pepper and blueberries may pop out more easily.

2. Use ground lamb for a different flavor.

3. Using your hands combine the ground turkey, olive oil, chopped mint, ground fennel, ground cumin, salt and pepper in a medium bowl.

4. Add the chopped red bell peppers, feta cheese and blueberries gently combining and then form into 6 equal burgers.

5. The blueberries or peppers may need to be popped back into the burgers.

6. Simply push them gently into place on the top side.

7. Season with additional salt and freshly ground black pepper.

8. Grill or pan fry over medium-high heat until the internal temperature reaches 166 °F and the meat is no longer pink in the center and the juices run clear.
9. Serve immediately.

Bones-to-Be Chicken Wingettes

Ingredients

- 2 tsps. Salt
- 2 serving All Purpose Low-Carb Baking Mix
- 4 2 oz., with bone Chicken Wing
- 2 tbsps. Chili Powder
- 2 tsp Red or Cayenne Pepper
- 2 tsps. Yellow Mustard Seed

Directions

1. Note: Use the Atkins recipe to make All Purpose Low-Carb Baking Mix for this recipe.
2. You will need half of a 1/5 cup = half of a serving.
3. Heat oven to 46 0°F.
4. Line a jelly-roll pan with foil, and spray with nonstick cooking spray.
5. Combine chili powder, 2 Tbsp.
6. baking mix, cayenne, mustard and salt in a large resealable bag.
7. Add half of the wingettes, and shake to coat.
8. Transfer to pan, and repeat with remaining wingettes.
9. Bake, turning occasionally, until crisp, browned and cooked through, 45 to 4 6 minutes.
10.   Transfer to a platter, and serve.

Mashed Cauliflower

Ingredients:

- 3 Oz. = Monterey Jack Cheese
- 3 Oz. = Cheddar Cheese
- Salt and Pepper to taste
- 2 Head = Cauliflower
- 6 Slices = Bacon
- 2 Oz. = Cream Cheese

Directions:

1. Cook the bacon and then crush.
2. inse and cut up the cauliflower.
3. Let some water to a boil and then include the cauliflower and boil for further 10 minutes.

4. As the cauliflower is boiling, dice the cheeses.
5. Strain the cauliflower.
6. Crush the cauliflower, and then put in the cream cheese and mash.
7. Add salt and pepper.
8. Mix in the cheese and bacon.
9. Shift to a baking plate and bake for 10 minutes at 4 6 0 degrees.

Chicken Soup With Dilled Mini-Matzo Balls

Ingredients

- 6 sprigs Parsley
- 2 oz. Dill
- 1/5 tsp leaf Dried Thyme Leaves
- 2 tsp Black Pepper
- 2 large Fresh fresh fresh eggs
- 2 tbsp. Canola Vegetable Oil
- 2 medium Scallions or Spring Fresh onion s
- 1/5 cup Matzo Meal
- 24 oz. boneless, cooked Chicken Thigh
- 4 14.6 oz. cans Chicken Broth, Bouillon or Consomme
- 4 2 cups Tap Water
- 2 small Red Fresh onion

21

- 6 small Carrots
- 2 stalk medium Celery
- 2 2 tsps. Garlic

Directions

1. For the soup: Combine chicken, broth, water, fresh onion , carrot, celery and garlic in a large saucepan.
2. Bring to a boil over high heat. Skim off foam that rises to surface.
3. Add parsley, dill, thyme and peppercorns; reduce heat to very low and simmer gently until flavors develop, about 2 2 hours.
4. Transfer chicken to a cutting board.

5. Strain broth into a clean container; skim off fat and season with salt and pepper to taste.
6. Discard solids.
7. Remove and discard skin from chicken; pull meat off bones and return to broth.
8. For the matzo balls: Combine fresh fresh fresh eggs , oil, dill and scallion in a small bowl.
9. Beat with a fork, then stir in matzo ball mix until well blended.
10. Cover and refrigerate for 16 minutes.
11. Meanwhile, bring a large pot of salted water to a boil over high heat.
12. With wet hands, shape matzo mixture into 16 balls using

2 level teaspoon for each, and drop balls into water.

13.   Reduce heat to low; cover and simmer until cooked through, about 16 minutes.

14.   Reheat soup.

15.   With a slotted spoon, transfer matzo balls to soup and serve.

Fresh Salmon Cakes With Avocado Tartar Sauce

Ingredients

- 2 tbsp. drained Capers
- 1/5 cup Parsley
- 2 large Fresh fresh fresh eggs
- 2 tsps. Old Bay Seasoning
- 2 tbsp. Fresh Fresh lemon Juice
- 2 tsps. fresh Dill
- 2 fruit without skin and seed California Avocado
- 16 oz. boneless Salmon
- 2 medium Red Sweet Pepper
- 2 stalk medium (8 -2 " - 8" long) Celery
- 2 tsp Original Stone Ground Mustard
- 6 tbsps. Real Mayonnaise

Directions

1. Preheat oven to 46 0°F.
2. Prepare a baking sheet with a small amount of oil in 4 spots about 6 inches apart. Set aside.
3. Coarsely chop the red pepper and celery.
4. Skin salmon if skin is intact and chop into 4-inch pieces.
5. Place all into a food processor.
6. A food processor is not required, just be sure to finely chop all ingredients before combining.
7. • Add the mustard, 2 tablespoons mayonnaise, capers, parsley, fresh fresh fresh eggs and Old Bay seasoning.
8. Pulse 4-6 times just until the salmon is chopped.

9. Season with salt and freshly ground black pepper.
10. Using a 3 cup measuring scoop - divide the mixture into 4 equal rounded mounds on the prepared baking sheet.
11. Cook for 25 minutes and move to serving plates.
12. Garnish each cake with 2 Tablespoons avocado tartar sauce.
13. Avocado Tartar Sauce: combine the avocado, 4 tablespoons mayonnaise, fresh lemon juice and chopped dill in a blender.
14. Blend until smooth adding salt and black pepper to taste.
15. 2 heaping tablespoons per serving.

Mini Italian Meatloaves

Ingredients

- 1/5 cup Dried Pine Nuts
- 2 large Fresh fresh fresh fresh eggs s
- 2 tsp Italian Seasoning
- 2 cups Spinach
- 2 2   oz. Spaghetti/Marinara Pasta Sauce
- 2 2 lbs. Ground Beef
- 12 oz. raw Italian Sausage
- 6 pieces Dried Porcini Mushrooms

Directions

1. Preheat oven to 4 6 0°F.
2. Mist 4 mini-loaf pans with olive-oil spray. Set aside.

3. Rehydrate mushrooms in 2 cup hot water, allow to sit for 10 minutes, then drain.
4. In a large mixing bowl, thoroughly combine ground beef seasoned with salt and freshly ground black pepper, chopped sausage, re-hydrated mushrooms, beaten fresh fresh fresh fresh eggs s , pine nuts, herbs and chopped spinach.
5. Divide into four equal portions and press into greased loaf pans.
6. Drizzle 2 tablespoon marinara sauce on top of each and place on a baking sheet.
7. Bake for 6 0 minutes.
8. Remove from oven and let rest for 10 minutes before serving.

Red Snapper, Vegetable And Pesto Packets

Ingredients

- 12 spear medium Asparagus
- 2 small Yellow Summer Squashes
- 2 tbsp. Fresh Fresh lemon Juice
- 2 small Red Sweet Pepper
- 2 tbsps. Pine Nuts
- 4 medium Scallions or Spring Fresh onion s
- 2 cup Pesto Sauce
- 2 tbsp. Extra Virgin Olive Oil
- 2 tsp Salt
- 2 2 lbs. Snapper

Directions

1. Heat oven to 426 °F.
2. Combine Basil Pesto, fresh lemon juice, olive oil and salt in a large bowl.
3. Gently spread half the mixture on fish, and toss vegetables with remaining mixture to coat.
4. Cut four 12 x 12 squares heavy-duty aluminum foil; fold each square in half, then open again.
5. Distribute vegetables evenly over one side of each square, leaving a 2 border; lay one fillet on top of each. Sprinkle with pine nuts.
6. Seal and crimp edges to make packets.
7. Transfer packets to a baking sheet, and bake 26 minutes.
8. Open packets directly on dinner plates.

Holiday Gingerbread

Ingredients

- 1/5 cup Unsalted Butter Stick
- 2 cup Heavy Cream
- 2 tsp Ginger
- 2 fl oz. Coffee
- 2 2   servings All Purpose Low-Carb Baking Mix
- 4 tbsps. Cocoa Powder
- 2 tsp Cinnamon
- 2 tsp Baking Powder 2 tsp Salt
- 1/5 tsp Cloves
- 2 tsp Nutmeg
- 2   cup 100% Stone Ground Whole Wheat Pastry Flour
- 10 tbsps. Sucralose Based Sweetener
- 8 large Fresh fresh fresh fresh eggs s

- 4 tsps. Ginger

Directions

1. Heat oven to 4 6 0°F.
2. Butter a 10 -inch round cake pan.
3. Whisk flour, 2 cup baking mix, cocoa powder, baking powder, salt, nutmeg, cinnamon, ground ginger and cloves in a bowl to combine.
4. In another bowl, beat fresh fresh fresh eggs yolks and sugar substitute with an electric mixer on high speed until thick ribbons form when the beaters are lifted, 4 to 4 minutes.
5. Beat in butter until smooth.
6. Add cream, fresh ginger and coffee; beat until thoroughly combined, about 2 minute.
7. With a clean mixing bowl and beaters, beat fresh fresh fresh eggs

whites until stiff peaks form, 4 to 4 minutes.

8. Mix one-third of fresh fresh fresh eggs whites into batter to lighten.

9. Gently fold in remaining fresh fresh fresh eggs whites in two additions until just combined.

10.   Pour batter into prepared pan.

11.   Bake until cake has risen and a toothpick inserted in the center comes out clean, 22- to 26 minutes.

12.   Cool cake in pan on a wire rack for 6 minutes.

13.   Remove cake from pan and let cool completely on the rack.

14.   If desired, whip extra cream flavored with ground ginger and sugar substitute to taste.

15.   Serve gingerbread with a dollop of flavored whipped cream.

Beef And Pepper Fajitas

Ingredients:

- 2 tbsp. of canola oil
- 2 sweet red pepper, thinly sliced
- 2 red fresh onion , thinly sliced
- 2 green sweet pepper, sliced thinly
- 1/8 cup of cilantro, fresh and chopped
- 12 tortillas, low carb
- ¾ cup of sour cream
- 2 ounce of lime, fresh
- 4 2 ounces of steak, boneless and thinly sliced
- 2 1 tsp. of garlic, minced
- 2 tsp. of salt
- 2 jalapeno pepper, seeded and chopped

- 2 tsp. of cumin, ground
- ¾ cup of green chile sauce
- 2 tbsp. of extra virgin olive oil

Directions:

1. First make the marinade.
2. To do this add the minced garlic, dash of salt, fresh lime juice, chopped jalapeno pepper, ground cumin and extra virgin olive oil to a large bowl.
3. Whisk until mixed.
4. Add the sliced steak to the marinade.
5. Toss well to coat.
6. Cover and place into the fridge to marinate for 2 hour.
7. After this time heat up the oven to 4 6 0 degrees.
8. Preheat an outdoor grill to medium or high heat.
9. While the oven and grill is heating up wrap the tortillas in a sheet of aluminum foil.

10. Remove the steak from the marinade.
11. Place onto the preheated grill and grill for 4 minutes on each side.
12. Remove and set aside.
13. Place a large skillet over medium to high heat.
14. Add in the canola oil and once the oil is heating up add in the sliced green and red peppers.
15. Add in the red fresh onion and stir well to mix.
16. Cook for 6 minutes or until the vegetables are soft.
17. Place the wrapped tortillas into the oven.
18. Warm for 16 minutes.
19. Serve the warm tortillas with the grilled steak and bell peppers.
20. Serve while piping hot.

Beef Fillet With Bacon And Gorgonzola Butter

Ingredients:

- 1/8 tsp. of salt
- 1/8 tsp. of black pepper
- 2 slices of bacon, thick cut
- 2 tsp. of extra virgin olive oil
- 8 ounces of mushroom caps, Portobello
- Scallions, chopped finely
- 2 tbsp. of unsalted butter

- 2 ounce of gorgonzola cheese
- 12 ounces of beef tenderloin, cut into small fillets

Directions:

1. Heat up the oven to 426 degrees.
2. While the oven is heating up add finely chopped scallions to a small bowl.
3. Add in the gorgonzola cheese and butter.
4. Stir well to mix.
5. Season the beef tenderloin with a dash of salt and black pepper.
6. Wrap a slice of bacon around the fillets.
7. Secure the bacon with a short toothpick.
8. Then place a large skillet over medium to high heat.
9. Add in the oil and once the oil is hot enough add in the beef tenderloin fillets.

10. Cook for 6 minutes on each side or until browned.
11. Transfer the beef tenderloin fillets to a large baking sheet.
12. Transfer to the oven to bake for 10 to 15 minutes.
13. Place the same skillet over medium to high heat.
14. Add in the mushrooms and season with a dash of salt and black pepper.
15. Reduce the heat to low and cook for 4 minutes or until the mushrooms are soft.
16. Serve the fillets with a dollop of the gorgonzola butter over the top.
17. Spoon the mushrooms on the side and serve.

Atkin's Diet Beef Stroganoff

Ingredients:

- 1 cup of fresh onion s, chopped
- 1/10 tsp. of black pepper
- 2 tbsp. of canola oil
- 2 tbsp. of unsalted butter
- 2 ounces of red wine
- 2 cup of beef broth
- 1/8 cup of sour cream
- 2 tsp. of Dijon mustard
- 1/10 tsp. of salt
- 4   ounces of mushrooms, cut into small pieces and stems
- 1, 25 -ounce beef skirt steak, trimmed and chopped into small pieces

Directions:

1. Season the skirt steak pieces with a dash of salt and black pepper.
2. Place a large skillet over medium to high heat.
3. Add in the canola oil and once the oil is hot enough add the steak pieces.
4. Cook for 2 minute on all sides.
5. Transfer the beef to a plate and set aside.
6. Add the butter into the skillet.
7. Once the butter is melted add in the chopped fresh onion .
8. Cook for 4 minutes or until soft.
9. Then add in the mushroom pieces and continue to cook for 10 minutes or until the liquid from the mushrooms fully evaporates.
10. Pour in the red wine.

11. Deglaze the bottom of the skillet and cook for 6 minutes.
12. Pour in the beef broth and cook for 10 minutes before adding in the sour cream and Dijon mustard.
13. Stir well to mix.
14. Add in the cooked meat and reduce the heat to low.
15. Allow to cook for5 to 10 minutes.
16. Season with a dash of salt and black pepper and remove from heat.
17. Serve while piping hot.

Check Lettuce Wraps With Peanut Sauce

Ingredients:

- 16 ounces of chicken, lean and ground
- 2 tbsp. of extra virgin olive oil
- 2 shallots, thinly sliced
- 2 green fresh onion s, fresh and thinly sliced
- 2 cloves of garlic, minced
- 8 leaves of butterhead lettuce
- 1/8 cup of water chestnuts
- 4 ounces of brown mushrooms
- 2 tbsp. of tamari
- 2 tbsp. of rice vinegar
- 2 tbsp. of sesame oil
- 2 tbsp. of peanut butter, creamy

- 2 packs of sweetener
- 2 tbsp. of water
- 2 tbsp. of Thai chili sauce, spicy

Directions:

1. Add the tamari, vinegar, sesame oil, creamy peanut butter, packs of sweetener, water and Thai chile sauce to a medium bowl.
2. Whisk to mix and heat in the microwave for 25 seconds.
3. Set aside.
4. Place a large skillet over medium heat.
5. Add in the ground chicken, minced garlic, thinly sliced shallots, sliced green fresh onion s and dash of salt and black pepper.
6. Stir to mix and cook for 10 to 15 minutes or until the chicken is cooked through.
7. Then add in the mushrooms and water chestnuts.

8. Stir well to mix. Continue to cook for an additional minute.

9. Add in the sauce mixture and stir well until coated.

10. Continue to cook for an additional5 to 10 minutes.

11. Remove from heat.

12. Spoon the chicken mixture into the lettuce leaves.

13. Serve immediately.

Burgundy Beef Stew

Ingredients:

- 2 stalk of celery, fresh and chopped
- 16 ounces of red wine
- 2, 14-ounce cans of beef broth
- 2 tsp. of bay leaf, crumbled
- 8 ounces of mushrooms, chopped into small pieces and stems
- 4 tsp. of thyme
- 2 tbsp. of parsley, fresh and chopped
- 4 ounces of bacon, thick cut
- 4 tbsp. of canola oil
- 1, 48-ounce beef chuck, trimmed, lean and cut into small pieces
- 2 cloves of garlic, minced

- 2 1 cups of fresh onion s, chopped
- • 3 cup of carrots, fresh and chopped

Ingredients for the baking mix:

- 1/10 cup of wheat bran
- 1 cup of soy flour, whole grain
- 1/5 cup of whey protein, vanilla
- 1/10 cup of flaxseed meal
- 1/8 cup of gluten flour, wheat

Directions:

1. First make the baking mix.
2. To do this add all of the ingredients to a large bowl.
3. Stir well to mix.
4. Remove 1/8 cup of the mixture and set the remaining mixture aside.

5. Cover the remaining mixture and store in a dark area.

6. Season the beef pieces with a dash of salt and black pepper.

7. Add the 1/8 cup of the baking mix to a bowl.

8. Add in the beef cubes and toss to coat until coated on all sides.

9. Place a large stock pot over medium heat.

10. Add in the bacon and cook for 6 to 8 minutes or until crispy.

11. Remove the bacon and place onto a large plate lined with paper towels to drain.

12. Once drained crumble the bacon and set aside.

13. Add the canola oil to the bacon fat in the stock pot.

14. Set over medium to high heat. Once the oil is hot enough add in the coated beef cubes.
15. Cook for 10 to 15 minutes or until browned.
16. Remove and set aside.
17. Add in the chopped fresh onion , chopped carrot and chopped celery.
18. Cook for 8 minutes or until soft.
19. Add in the minced garlic and cook for an additional minute.
20. Pour in the red wine and deglaze the pan.
21. Increase the heat of the stove to high.
22. Bring the wine to a boil and allow to boil until it's reduced to at least one cup.

23. This should take at least 6 minutes.
24. Then pour in the beef broth and the bay leaf.
25. Add the cooked beef cubes back into the pot.
26. Reduce the heat to low and cover.
27. Allow to simmer for 2 hours.
28. After this time add in the chopped mushrooms, chopped thyme and chopped parsley.
29. Stir to mix and continue to cook for an additional 45 minutes or until the beef is soft.
30. Remove the bay leaf and remove from heat.
31. Serve the stew with the crumbled bacon over the top as a garnish.

Cajun Black Salmon With A Fresh Cucumber Relish

Ingredients:

- 2 pack of sweetener
- 12 ounces of cauliflower, fresh and chopped
- 1 tsp. of basil, dried
- 2 tbsp. of paprika, smoked
- 1 tsp. of oregano
- 1/8 tsp. of cayenne pepper
- 2, 12 ounces of salmon, boneless
- 2 tbsp. of extra virgin olive oil
- ¾ tsp. of salt
- 1 of a cucumber, chopped into small piece
- 2 lime, fresh and juice only
- 2 tbsp. of dill, fresh

- 2 tbsp. of thyme, fresh

Directions:

1. Set a medium saucepan over medium to high heat.
2. Add in 4 cups of water and bring the water to a boil.
3. While the water is coming to a boil add the cucumber pieces to a medium bowl.
4. Add in the lime juice and toss well to mix.
5. Set aside.
6. Then make the relish.
7. To do this add in the sweetener, fresh dill, spoonful of the extra virgin olive oil and a dash of salt and black pepper.
8. Stir well to mix.

9. Then make the rub. To do this add the basil, smoked paprika, oregano, cayenne pepper, thyme and dash of salt to a small bowl.

10. Stir well to mix.

11. Add the cauliflower to the boiling water.

12. Allow to cook for 10 minutes or until soft.

13. After this time drain the cauliflower and set aside to keep warm.

14. Pat the salmon fillets dry with a few paper towels.

15. Brush the salmon with the olive oil until coated on all sides.

16. Rub the rub over the surface of the salmon.

17. Place a large skillet over medium to high heat.

18. Add in a spoonful of the olive oil. Once the oil is hot enough add in the seasoned salmon fillets.

19. Cook for 5 to 10 minutes on each side or until black.

20. Mash the cauliflower finely and coat with one tablespoon of the olive oil.

21. Season with a dash of salt and black pepper.

22. Stir to mix and spoon onto two large serving plates.

23. Serve with the black salmon and cucumber relish garnished over the top.

Cajun Spiced Pork Chops

Ingredients:

- 1 tsp. of garlic, powdered
- 1 tsp. of cayenne pepper
- 1, 24-ounce pork chop, raw with the bone
- 1 tbsp. of butter, unsalted
- 1 tbsp. of vegetable oil
- 2 tbsp. of paprika, smoked
- 1 tsp. of cumin
- 1 tsp. of sage, ground
- 1 tsp. of black pepper

Directions:

1. Add the smoked paprika, ground cumin, ground sage, black pepper, powdered garlic and cayenne pepper to a large shallow plate.
2. Stir well to mix.
3. Season the pork chops with a dash of salt.
4. Place into the plate and dredge on both sides evenly.
5. Place a large skillet over high heat.
6. Add in the butter and vegetable oil.
7. Stir to mix and once the butter is melted add in the pork chop.
8. Cook for 10 to 15 minutes or until cooked through on all sides.

4. Remove and serve immediately.

Green Fresh Onion And Cheddar Cheese Pie

Ingredients:

- 1 tsp. of salt
- 1/8 tsp. of black pepper
- 1/8 tsp. of Tabasco sauce
- 1, 8-ounce pie crust, premade
- 4 fresh fresh fresh fresh eggs s , large and whole
- 1/5 cup of heavy whipping cream
- 4   cups of cheddar cheese, shredded
- 6 scallions, thinly sliced

Directions:

1. Bake the pie crust according to the directions on the package.
2. Heat up the oven to 4 6 0 degrees.

3. While the oven is heating up place a medium saucepan over low heat.
4. Add in the large fresh fresh fresh fresh eggs s , heavy whipping cream, shredded cheese and sliced green fresh onion s.
5. Stir well until mixed.
6. Cook for 8 minutes or until the cheese is melted.
7. Season the mix with a dash of salt, black pepper and Tabasco sauce.
8. Pour this mixture into the prebaked pie crust.
9. Place into the oven to bake for 45 minutes or until the filling set.
10. Remove and serve while warm.

Easy Cheese Soufflés

Ingredients:

- 1/10   cup of pastry flour, whole wheat and ground
- ¾ cup of heavy cream
- ¾ cup of water
- 2 cups of cheddar cheese, shredded
- 1/8 tsp. of salt
- 1/10 tsp. of cayenne pepper
- 1/8 cup of parmesan cheese, grated
- 6 fresh fresh fresh fresh eggs s , large and whole
- 1/8 cup of butter, unsalted
- 2 tbsp. of soy flour, whole rain

Directions:

1.   Heat up the oven to 4 6 0 degrees.

2. While the oven is heating up grease two large soufflé dishes with cooking spray.

3. In the soufflé dishes sprinkle two spoonfuls of grated parmesan cheese into the dish.

4. Then add the fresh fresh fresh eggs yolks into a small bowl.

5. Add the fresh fresh fresh eggs whites into a separate bowl. Set aside.

6. Place a medium saucepan over medium heat.

7. Add in the butter and once the butter is melted add in the soy and pastry flour.

8. Add in the heavy cream and water.

9. Whisk to mix.

10. Add in the remaining Parmesan cheese, shredded cheddar cheese, dash of salt and cayenne pepper.
11. Stir well to mix.
12. Bring this mixture to a boil.
13. Whisk until smooth in consistency.
14. Remove this mixture from heat.
15. Add in the fresh fresh fresh eggs yolks and stir well to mix.
16. Transfer this mixture to a large bowl and set aside for later use.
17. Use an electric mixer and beat the fresh fresh fresh eggs whites on the highest setting until peaks begin to form.
18. Fold the fresh fresh fresh eggs whites into the cheese mixture until fully incorporated.
19. Pour the soufflé mixture into the prepared soufflé dishes.

20. Place into the oven to bake for 40 to 46 minutes or until completely baked through.
21. Remove and allow to cool for 10 to 16 minutes before serving.

Hearty Chicken, Sage And Ham Soup

Ingredients:

- 16 ounces of chicken breasts, boneless and fully cooked
- 2 tsp. of sage, ground
- 4 ounces of ham, fresh and fully cooked
- 1 tsp. of black pepper
- 1 tsp. of salt
- 2 fresh lemon , fresh, 2 tsp. of zest and 2 tsp. of juice
- 2 tbsp. of extra virgin olive oil
- 2 tbsp. of shallots, thinly sliced
- 2, 142 -ounce cans of chicken broth
- 2 cup of water

Directions:

1. Place a large saucepan over medium heat.
2. Add in the extra virgin olive oil and once the oil is hot enough add in the sliced shallots.
3. Cook for 2 minute or until soft.
4. Add in the cans of chicken broth, water and cooked chicken, cooked ham and ground sage.
5. Stir well to mix.
6. Bring the mixture to a boil.
7. Once boiling reduce the heat to low.
8. Cook at a simmer for 6 minutes.
9. Add in the fresh fresh lemon zest and fresh fresh lemon juice.
10. Stir to incorporate.
11. Season the mixture with a dash of salt and black pepper.

12. Continue to cook for5 to 10 minutes.
13. Remove from heat and serve immediately.

Cheese And Chard Casserole

Ingredients:

- 2 1 cups of muenster cheese, shredded
- 1 cup of parmesan cheese, freshly grated
- 2 tbsp. of extra virgin olive oil
- ¾ pound of swiss chard

- 2 sweet red pepper, chopped
- 2 fresh onion , thinly sliced
- 1 tsp. of salt
- 1/8 tsp. of black pepper

Directions:

1. First heat up the oven to 4 6 0 degrees.
2. While the oven is heating up grease a large baking dish with some cooking spray.
3. Place a large Dutch oven over medium to high heat.
4. Add in one spoonful of the extra virgin olive oil.
5. Once the oil is hot enough add in the swiss chard.
6. Cook for 4 to 4 minutes or until wilted.
7. Transfer into a colander and drain.

8. Squeeze out the excess liquid.

9. Place a large skillet over medium heat.

10. Add in the remaining extra virgin olive oil.

11. Once the oil is hot enough add in the sweet red pepper and fresh onion .

12. Cook for 8 minutes or until soft.

13. Add the chard back into the skillet and toss to coat.

14. Season with a dash of salt and black pepper.

15. Add in the muenster cheese and stir well to mix.

16. Spoon this mixture into the prepared baking dish.

17. Sprinkle the grated parmesan cheese over the top.

18. Cover the baking dish with a sheet of aluminum foil.
19. Place into the oven to bake for 4 6 minutes.
20. After this time remove the sheet of aluminum foil.
21. Continue to bake for an additional 10 minutes or until the cheese is bubbly.
22. Remove and cool for 10 to 16 minutes before serving.

Chicken Breasts Smothered In Tarragon Cream Sauce

Ingredients:

- 2 tbsp. of mustard, Dijon
- ¾ tsp. of tarragon
- 1/10 tsp. of salt
- 1/10 tsp. of black pepper
- 4 6 ounces of chicken breasts, boneless and bone removed
- 2 tbsp. of butter, unsalted
- 2 tbsp. of canola oil
- 1 cup of heavy cream

Directions:

1. Season the chicken breasts with a dash of salt and black pepper.
2. Place a large skillet over medium heat.
3. Add in the butter and canola oil.
4. Once the butter is melted add in the chicken.
5. Cook for 10 to 16 minutes or until browned on all sides.
6. Then reduce the heat to low.
7. Continue to cook for an additional 16 minutes or until the chicken is fully cooked through.
8. Remove and transfer to a large plate.
9. Add in the Dijon mustard and tarragon.

10. Continue to cook for 6 minutes or until the sauce is thick in consistency.
11. Season the mixture with a dash of salt and black pepper.
12. Pour the sauce over the chicken and serve immediately.

Soup With Pork And Fennel

INGREDIENTS

- 2 cloves of garlic, chopped into quarters
- tsp salt
- 1 tsp ground white pepper
- cups of water
- cup chicken stock

- 2 cup of fat cream
- 46 0 g pork neck
- 46 0 g of cauliflower chopped into flowers
- 280 g sliced fresh fennel

PREPARATION

1. Put all the ingredients except the cream in a slow cooker.

2. Cook at high temperature for 6 hours.

3. Remove the pork from the soup and chop. Set aside.

4. Beat the soup with a blender until smooth.

5. Add cream and minced pork.

6. Try it and, if necessary, add extra salt and pepper.

Creamy Cheese Soup With Broccoli

INGREDIENTS

- 4 tbsp Dijon mustard
- 0.6 tsp cayenne pepper
- tsp dried tarragon leaves
- 284 g minced broccoli
- 284 g grated cauliflower

- 4 4 10 g grated cheddar cheese

- 2 cloves of chopped garlic
- 2 tbsp butter
- 24 8 g buttercream
- 26 0 g unsweetened almond milk
- 1.44kg of chicken stock
- 0.6 tsp salt

PREPARATION

1. Sauté the garlic in melted butter in a large saucepan over medium heat until golden brown.

2. Add cream, milk, chicken stock, salt, mustard, cayenne pepper, and tarragon. Bring to a boil.

3. Add chopped broccoli and cauliflower.

4. Bring to a boil.

5. Reduce heat to a minimum and cook for about 6 -10 minutes, stirring occasionally.

6. Add the cheese and simmer until the cheese melts.

Low Carb Chicken Noodle Soup

INGREDIENTS

- 8 stalks of celery, chopped
- l chicken bone broth
- 46 0 g pre-cooked and chopped chicken
- 4 tsp fresh chopped basil
- 4 tsp fresh chopped parsley
- 0.6 tsp sea salt
- bay leaves

- 46 6 g zucchini chopped with spirals

- 4 tbsp coconut oil
- 4 minced cloves of garlic

- chopped fresh onion
- 0.6 tsp ground turmeric
- 2 medium turnip, diced

PREPARATION

1. Heat 2 tablespoon of coconut oil in a saucepan over medium heat.

2. Add garlic and fry until fragrant.

3. Add fresh onion s and turmeric.

4. Cook until fresh onion is clear.

5. Add turnips and celery with the remaining 2 tablespoons of coconut oil.

6. Cook for about 10 minutes.

7. Add the broth, chicken, basil, parsley, salt, and bay leaf.

8. Bring to a boil, then reduce heat.

9. Cover and simmer for about 40 minutes.

10.   Remove from heat.

11.   Remove the bay leaf.

12.   Add the spiralized zucchini and cover the pan.

13.   Leave to brew for 10 minutes to soften the zucchini noodles.

Creamy Salmon Soup With Coconut Milk

INGREDIENTS

- 2 green chopped fresh onion s
- 10 08 g chicken bone broth
- 2 tbsp lard or coconut oil
- 2 small chopped fresh onion
- 4 minced cloves of garlic
- 2 medium turnips, peeled and diced
- 2 medium carrots, chopped
- 4 stalks of celery, chopped
- 2 tbsp cider vinegar
- 6 sprigs of fresh thyme, chopped
- 0.6 tsp sea salt
- 46 6 g sliced salmon fillet
- 425 g canned coconut milk
- 2 tbsp lime juice or fresh lemon juice

PREPARATION

1. Melt lard or coconut oil in a large saucepan.

2. Sauté the fresh onion until transparent.

3. Add the garlic and continue to simmer until fragrant.

4. Then add turnips, carrots, and celery.

5. Cook for another 6 -10 minutes until the vegetables are lightly browned.

6. Add the broth, vinegar, thyme, and salt.

7. Reduce heat, cover, and simmer for 45 minutes to soften vegetables.

8. Put 2 cups of soup in a blender and beat everything until smooth.

9. Add mashed potatoes to the remaining soup.

10. Add salmon and coconut milk, and continue cooking until the fish is cooked.

11. Season with lime juice and garnish with green fresh onion s.

Creamy Cheese Soup With Broccoli

INGREDIENTS

- Salt and pepper to taste
- 1 tsp xanthan gum
- 1 cup chicken stock
- 2 cup chopped broccoli
- 2 cup of fat cream

- 2 1 cup grated cheddar cheese

- 2 tbsp butter
- 2 chopped small fresh onion
- 2 medium chopped garlic cloves

PREPARATION

1. Preheat the pan on the stove.

2. Put fresh onion , chopped garlic, salt, pepper, and oil in it and cook over medium heat until soft.

3. Add xanthan gum and chicken stock. Mix well.

4. Put the broccoli in the pan and make sure it is covered with the stock.

5. Quickly add cream.

6. Bring the soup to a boil, stirring often.

7. Slowly start adding cheese, stirring again.

8. Serve with plenty of broccoli and cheese.

Ginger Pumpkin Soup

INGREDIENTS

- 2 small fresh onion
- 0.6 l vegetable stock
- 8 g fresh ginger
- 2.46 g of salt

- 2.46 g black pepper

- 2 small pumpkin
- 44.4 6 g of olive oil
- 2 clove of garlic

PREPARATION

1. Cut the pumpkin in half and pull out the core.

2. Trim the tail and pull out the seeds, and cut the pumpkin into cubes.

3. In a large saucepan, heat 2 tbsp.

4. olive oil.

5. Add fresh onion s and garlic, and cook until tender, stirring frequently.

6. Add pumpkin and ginger, and cook for 2-4 minutes.

7. Add vegetable stock and bring to a boil.

8. Season with salt and pepper.

9. Cook over low heat for 4 6 –40 minutes until the pumpkin is soft.

10. Using a hand blender, beat the soup until smooth.

11. Serve with whipped cream.

Creamy Cheese Soup With Vegetables

INGREDIENTS

- 2 tsp pepper
- 1/10 tsp nutmeg
- 2 cups chicken or beef broth
- 2 small spinach
- 2 cup fat cream
- 114 g Cheddar Cheese

- 114 g gouda cheese
- 2 cups broccoli
- 2 medium carrot
- 2 small fresh onion
- 2 tbsp olive oil
- 2 tsp garlic powder
- 5 tsp salt

PREPARATION

1. Add olive oil to a large saucepan and put on medium heat.

2. Add chopped carrots and fresh onion s, mix well and cook for 1-2 minutes.

3. Add garlic, broccoli, seasoning, and spices.

4. Mix and cook for another 2 minute.

5. Add bone broth, mix and cook for 8-10 minutes until the vegetables are soft.

6. Turn off the heat and mix with heavy cream.

7. Pour 2 of the soup mixture into the blender, add the spinach and beat until smooth.

8. You can mix the whole soup if you prefer a completely thick consistency.

9. Return the contents of the blender to a large pan and mix with two kinds of cheese until they are completely melted.

10. Season to taste and sprinkle with broccoli and cheese if desired.

Spicy Sausage And Pepper Soup

INGREDIENTS

- 2 cup jalapeno tomatoes
- 2 cups beef
- 2 teaspoons chili powder
- 2 teaspoons of caraway seeds
- 2 teaspoons minced garlic
- 2 teaspoon Italian seasoning

- 1 teaspoon kosher salt

- 64 6 g spicy Italian sausages
- 6 cups raw spinach
- 2 medium green bell pepper
- 2 medium red bell pepper
- 1 medium fresh onion

PREPARATION

1. Cut the sausage and sauté it.

2. Add chopped peppers, tomatoes, beef, and spices to the pan.

3. Add the sausage on top and mix well.

4. Sauté your fresh onion s and garlic to a translucent state and add to the pan.

5. Top with spinach and cook for 4 hours.

6. After 4 hours, mix, reduce heat, and simmer another 2 hours.

Soup With Red Pepper And Cauliflower

INGREDIENTS

- 4 medium green fresh onion s, diced
- 4 cups chicken stock
- 2 cup fat cream
- 2 tsp garlic powder
- 2 tsp dried thyme
- 2 tsp smoked paprika
- 1/5 tsp red pepper
- 114 g goat cheese

- Salt and pepper to taste

- 2 red bell peppers
- 2 head of cauliflower
- 6 tbsp duck fat

PREPARATION

1. Cut the bell pepper in half and peel the seeds.

2. Bake for 10-16 minutes or until the skin is charred and blackened.

3. Once the pepper is ready, remove it from the oven and place it in a container with a lid or bag for storing food.

4. Let the pepper steam to make it softer.

5. Cut the cauliflower into inflorescences and season with 2 tbsp.

6. molten duck fat, salt, and pepper.

7. Bake cabbage for 4 0-4 6 minutes at 25 0 degrees.

8. Remove the peel from the pepper by thoroughly cleaning it.

9. Pour 4 tbsp into the pan. duck fat.

10.   When it heats, add the cubes of green fresh onion s, seasoning, chicken stock, red pepper, and cabbage.

11.   Cook for 10-25 minutes.

12.   Mix everything well with a blender, then add cream and mix again.

13.   Serve with crispy bacon and goat cheese.

14. Garnish with thyme and green fresh onion s.

Spicy Low-Carb Spinach Soup

INGREDIENTS

- 100 ml of coconut milk
- 2 hot water
- 2 large bag of washed spinach

- Soy sauce

- 2 teaspoon fresh ginger
- 2 clove of garlic

PREPARATION

1. Cook 2 teaspoon of raw 2 in oil in a soup pot for 2 minute.

2. Stir in a piece of garlic for 2 minutes.

105

3. Pour and crush 100 ml coconut milk and 4 60 ml water

4. Take a broth tablet with you

5. Cook with a pan lid.

6. Put the spinach in a spoon

7. Cook for 2-4 minutes.

8. Cut the spinach leaves into slices.

9. Grate the soup with a hand mixer or food processor,

10. Season to taste with soy sauce.

11. Decorate the soup with spinach bars and red thread

Creamy Zucchini Soup With Salmon Chips

INGREDIENTS

- 126 ml fresh whipped cream
- Salt and pepper
- 150 grams of smoked salmon chips
- 2 clove of garlic
- 2 courgettes
- 2 vegetable stock cubes
- 1-liter water

PREPARATION

1. Cut the fresh onion , garlic, and dice the zucchini.

2. Heat olive oil a little in a soup pan and fry fresh onion s and garlic until it becomes glassy.

3. Add zucchini cubes and cook for another 4 minutes on high heat.

4. Add 2 liter of water to the stock cube and bring it to a boil.

5. Boil at low temperature for 8 minutes.

6. Puree the soup with a hand blender and stir in the whipped cream. Season with salt and pepper.

7. Divide the soup into plates and add the appropriate amount of salmon chips.

8. You can also heat the salmon for another minute.

Pumpkin Soup With Coconut And Curry

INGREDIENTS

- v salt and pepper
- 425 ml chicken broth
- 425 ml of water

- 25 0 ml of coconut milk

- 800 grams sliced pumpkin cubes
- 1-2 cloves of garlic
- 2 tsp curry powder

PREPARATION

1. Melt a piece of butter in a large soup pot.

2. Heat the chicken broth in another pan at the same time.

3. Cut the fresh onion into small pieces and fry gently in the pan for 6 minutes.

4. Add the diced pumpkin and fry it until softer.

5. Add the garlic, curry powder, salt, and pepper to the fresh onion and cook together for 2 minute.

6. Simultaneously heat the coconut milk in a separate pan and stir in occasionally.

7. Add the chicken stock and water to the whole and mix well.

8. Lower your gas burner to a lower position.

9. Boil slowly for 25 minutes and stir occasionally.

10. Put the soup in the blender together with the coconut milk and mix until smooth.

11. Then add it to the soup pan again and heat it until it is warm enough to be served.

Moroccan Style Chickpea Soup

INGREDIENTS

- 2 tablespoons chopped fresh parsley.

- 2 tablespoon turmeric.
- 2 tablespoon of cinnamon coffee
- 2 tablespoons grated fresh ginger coffee.
- A few strands of saffron.
- 4 tablespoons olive oil.
- A nip of sea salt and black pepper.

- Half grated zucchini with spiralizer.

- 4 ripe tomatoes, chopped
- 26 0 g of cooked chickpeas.
- 2 chopped fresh onion .
- 2 branch of chopped celery.
- 2 chicken thighs
- 2 tablespoons chopped fresh cilantro.

PREPARATION

1. We marinate chicken thighs with cinnamon and turmeric.

2. In a deep casserole, sauté chicken thighs in olive oil and brown them for about 4 -4 minutes.

3. Then add the chopped fresh onion and grated ginger.

4. We stir well.

5. Add the celery, parsley, and cilantro.

6. Sauté the whole over medium heat for a few minutes.

7. Next, we remove the chicken thighs and reserve them.

8. Add the chopped tomatoes and a tablespoon of olive oil to the casserole.

9. In a cup of hot water, we soak the saffron threads.

10. Then add the saffron along with the water to the casserole.

11. Then add the chicken and three more cups of hot water.

12. Add the salt and pepper.

13. Cover the casserole and let the whole cook for half an hour, stirring occasionally.

14. Remove the chicken from the casserole, remove the bones, and add the shredded meat back to the casserole.

15. Finally, we incorporate the chickpeas.

16. Prepare the "spaghetti" zucchini with the spiralizer.

Nopal Soup

INGREDIENTS

- 2 cloves of garlic
- 2 chipotle chili in adobo
- 4 cups of vegetable stock
- 2 tablespoon dried oregano

- Salt and pepper to taste

- 2 pounds of nopales, clean and diced
- 4 Roma tomatoes
- 1/8 white fresh onion

OPTIONAL COVERAGES

- Chives

- Fresh lemon or Lime Juice

- Avocado

- Coriander

PREPARATION

1. Cook the nopales for 25 -26 minutes in boiling water with salt or until they lose their bright color and are tender to bit.

2. Place the tomatoes, fresh onion , garlic, and chipotle in a blender glass.

3. Blend until you get a creamy consistency.

4. Remove the nopales from the heat, drain them, and rinse them with enough cold water. Leave aside.

5. In a pot, sauté the tomato sauce for about 4 minutes.

6. Add cooked nopales and oregano to tomato broth.

7. Let cook another 16 minutes.

8. Add salt and pepper to taste.

9. Serve on soup plates and add toppings.

Matzo Ball Soup

INGREDIENTS

MATZO BALLS

- 2 medium yellow fresh onion , chopped
- 1/8 cup of Coconut Aminos
- 1 teaspoon freshly ground black pepper
- 6 medium carrots, peeled and sliced
- 4 celery stalks, diced
- 2 parsnips, peeled and sliced
- 2 cup fresh parsley, chopped

- 8 cups of vegetable broth without sodium

- COVER

- 4 tablespoons fresh dill, finely chopped

- 2 1 cups quinoa flakes
- 2 1 cups of mixture gluten purpose flour
- 2 teaspoons fresh onion powder
- 2 teaspoon garlic powder
- 1/8 teaspoon of sea salt
- 2 cups of boiling water

- 6 tablespoons pumpkin puree

- SOUP

PREPARATION

1. Preheat the oven to 25 0-4 00 degrees F.

2. Cover a 16 x 14 inch baking sheet with parchment paper.

3. To make matzo balls: Beat quinoa flakes, flour, fresh onion powder, garlic powder, and salt in a medium bowl.

4. Add the boiling water and the pumpkin and stir to combine.

5. Take at least a tablespoon of the mixture and form a ball.

6. Place the ball on the prepared baking sheet. Repeat until you have used the entire mixture.

7. You should have approximately 45 balls.

8. Bake the matzo balls until they are a light golden color, approximately 25 minutes.

9. Turn the balls halfway through cooking.

10.   Transfer the baking sheet from the oven to a wire rack and let it stand for 10 minutes.

11.   To make the soup: heat the fresh onion in a large pot over medium heat and stir until it begins to release its aroma, approximately for a minute.

12.   Add the Coconut Aminos, black pepper, carrots, celery, parsnips, and parsley and cook,   stirring occasionally,   until   the   vegetables

release their aroma and are slightly soft, about two minutes.

13. Add the broth and boil.

14. Reduce the heat intensity, cover the pot, and let simmer for about 4 6 minutes.

15. Serve immediately and place several matzo balls in each bowl of soup.

16. Sprinkle dill in the soup.

17. The soup tastes even better the next day, and even better two days later.

Vegetable Broth Without Sodium

INGREDIENTS

- 4 celery stalks, sliced
- 6 sprigs of dill
- 4 sprigs of parsley
- 4 scallions

- 10 cups of water

- 2 yellow fresh onion s, sliced
- 4 cloves garlic, minced
- 6 carrots, peeled and sliced

PREPARATION

1. Add the fresh onion s over medium heat to a large pot and stir until the scent is released, about a minute.

2. Add the garlic, carrots, celery, dill, parsley, and scallions and cook for about a minute until the herbs release their fragrance.

3. Add the water and allow it to boil.

4. Low the heat, cover the pot, and cook for 46 minutes.

5. Turn off the heat and allow about 16 minutes to cool the broth.

6. Filter the broth through a sieve and freeze it into ice buckets, or pour it into glass jars if you use it immediately.

7. It's going to stay a week or so.

Comforting Noodle And Chickpea Soup

INGREDIENTS

- fresh cilantro chopped to taste
- 2 cup fresh onion , diced
- 2 carrots, sliced
- 2 celery stalk, diced
- 2 medium diced potatoes
- 4 cloves garlic, minced
- 1 teaspoon dried thyme
- 4 cups of vegetable stock
- 2 cups of water
- 1/8 cup chicken seasoning

- 6 ounces cooked spaghetti 2 cups cooked chickpeas
- Salt and pepper to taste

DRESSING FOR "CHICKEN"

- 11 tablespoon dried basil
- 2 teaspoon oregano
- 1 teaspoon of turmeric
- 2 teaspoons sea salt
- *2 ⅓ cup nutritional yeast*
- 4 tablespoons fresh onion powder
- 2 tablespoon garlic powder

PREPARATION

1. Sauté the fresh onion in a medium saucepan over medium heat until it begins to soften, about 4 minutes.

2. Add the carrots, potatoes, and celery and sauté for 2-4 minutes.

3. Add garlic, thyme, "chicken seasoning," vegetable stock, and water.

4. Cook over medium-low heat until all vegetables are tender, about 25 minutes.

5. Add the chickpeas and pasta.

6. Season with salt and pepper to taste.

7. Serve with some fresh cilantro on top.

Soup Loaded With Miso Noodles

INGREDIENTS

- 2 cup julienne zucchini
- 2 cup thinly sliced shiitake mushrooms
- 2 cup broccoli corsages
- 4 tablespoons miso paste
- 2 package of firm tofu
- , cut into one-inch cubes
- 1/8 cup chopped green fresh onion

- 2 sheet of roasted nori seaweed, cut into pieces

- 4 servings of buckwheat noodles or brown rice noodles, uncooked
- 4 cups of vegetable stock

- 4 cups of water
- 2 cup of carrot cut into julienne

PREPARATION

- Prepare the noodles as per the instructions for the box.

- Set them apart.

- Cook the vegetable stock and water in a medium saucepan over high heat.

- Remove the carrots, courgettes, mushrooms, and broccoli, add heat and cook for five minutes.

- Use a ladle to pass to a small bowl a cup of broth.

- Use a fork in the broth to dissolve the miso paste and return it to the pot.

- Add tofu, green fresh onion s, and cooked noodles and cook for another minute until warm.

- Move to bowls and cover with seaweed nori.

Bone Mineral Broth And Vegetables

INGREDIENTS

- small bunch of celery, including the heart, cut into pieces
- 6 cloves of unpeeled garlic, cut in half
- 2 normal or small winter squash with peel, seeded and cut into pieces

- 2 piece of fresh ginger 6 inches, sliced
- 4 cups chopped vegetables, such as kale or chard
- 1 bunch fresh parsley
- 2 package of 40 g dried daikon radish 2 strips of 6 inchesof dried Kombu seaweed
- 6 mushroom shiitake dry
- 6 carrots cut into pieces
- 2 medium fresh onion s cut into pieces
- 2 leek, with white and green parts, cut into pieces

PREPARATION

1. Combine all ingredients in a broth or large soup pot.

2. Fill the pot 2 inches below the edge with water, cover it and let it boil.

3. Remove the lid, reduce the temperature to medium/low, and let it boil for a minimum of two hours.

4. As the broth heats up, some of the water will evaporate; add more if the vegetables are exposed.

5. Cook over low heat until you can taste the delicacy of vegetables.

6. Strain the broth and pour it into glass jars.

7. Refrigeration works well with any broth.

Noodle Soup With Broccoli And Ginger

INGREDIENTS

- ¾ cup wheat-free or regular tamari
- 2 medium fresh onion s, diced 4 tablespoons fresh ginger root, chopped or finely grated
- 4 tablespoons mirin
- 6 medium carrots, diced

- 4 medium parsnips, diced

- 4 medium broccoli heads
- 2 package of small rice noodles
- 16 ounces firm tofu, cut into 1/8 to 1 inch cubes
- 2 pieces of two inches of wakame or alaria seaweed

135

- 4 quarts of water

PREPARATION

1. Separate the broccoli stems from their heads.

2. Remove the hard outer layer of the stems and cut them into small bite-sized pieces.

3. Set them aside.

4. Separate broccoli headed into small pieces and set aside.

5. Cook the noodles, strain them and let them cool.

6. Set them aside.

7. Sauté the tofu in a nonstick skillet for 4 to 4 minutes.

8. Add 4 teaspoons of tamari and sauté for another 4 to 4 minutes.

9. Set it aside.

10. Place the wakame or alaria seaweed in 4 liters of water and bring it to a boil.

11. Lower the heat to medium, add the fresh onion s and cook for 10 minutes.

12. Remove the vegetables from the sea, cut them into small pieces, and return them to the pot.

13. Add the ginger, the remaining tamari, and the peeper.

14. Continue cooking over medium heat for 6 minutes.

15. Add carrots, parsnips, and broccoli stems.

16. Cook for 2 minutes.

17. Gently stir the noodles and sauteed tofu. Cook for 2 minute.

18. Add the broccoli heads.

19. Cook over low heat until the broccoli is tender, for about 2 or 4 minutes.

Pancakes With Berries & Whipped Cream

INGREDIENTS

- 25 ml of cream double

- 2 fresh fresh fresh fresh eggs s
- 2 tablespoons cream cheese
- 1/8 teaspoon sweetener
- 2 pinch of cinnamon
- 40 g blueberries

PREPARATION

1. Mix fresh fresh fresh fresh eggs s ,
   cream cheese, sweetener and
   cinnamon to a dough.

2. Stir the ingredients until you have a smooth dough.

3. Let the mass rest for 2 minutes to allow the bubbles to settle.

4. Put half of the dough in a hot non-stick skillet that has been greased with butter.

5. Fry the dough for 4 - 4 minutes over medium heat until it is golden brown, then turn over and fry for 4 minutes on the other side.

6. Repeat this with the rest of the dough.

7. Beat the crème double until it is firm and serve the pancakes with the crème and blueberries.

Grilled Lamb And Child With Mint Salad And Feta Cheese

COMPONENT PART

- Lamb fillet 150 grams
- 100 grams fresh fresh fresh eggs plant sliced vertically
- 2 tbsp of mint, chopped
- 2 tsp dill, fresh
- 40 grams of ground feta cheese
- Handful of spinach

- 2 tbsp fresh lemon juice

- 2 tbsp olive oil
- 2 tbsp red wine vinegar
- 2 tbsp fresh oregano
- 1/5 teaspoon salt
- 1/5 tbsp black pepper pepper

PREPARATION

1. Put oil, add vinegar, add oregano, some little salt and pepper, and fatty mutton and cubs.

2. Bake 6-8 lambs in a warm frying pan or grill on one side until the baked children turn dark gold.

3. Put half mint, dill, spinach, and feta cheese on a plate.

4. Cut the lamb into thick slices and divide it into plates of fresh fresh fresh eggs plant.

5. Garnish with the remaining feta cheese and pour the fresh lemon juice into the lamb.

Stuffed Veal Chop

INGREDIENT

- 60 g Roquefort cheese
- 2 veal chop
- 100 ml white wine
- 100 ml of soy cream

- 1 fresh lemon

- 2 fresh onion s
- 2 garlic cloves
- 2 pear salt, pepper
- 2 pinch cane sugar
- 2 tbsp olive oil
- 2 stems marjoram

PREPARATION

1. Peel the fresh onion s and cut into 6 mm thick rings.

2. Peel and crush garlic cloves.

3. Wash the pear, quarter and remove the core.

4. Halve pear quarter.

5. Put the fresh onion rings, garlic and pear pieces in a roasting pan and season with salt, pepper, and sugar, drizzle with 2 tablespoon of olive oil.

6. Bake in the preheated oven at 25 0 ° C for about 10 minutes.

7. Wash the marjoram, shake dry, pluck the leaves, and chop.

8. Crumble Roquefort and mix with marjoram.

9. Cut a bag horizontally into the meat and fill with the cheese; put the incision with 2 wooden skewers.

10. Salt and pepper the meat.

11. Heat the remaining oil in a heavy pan and fry the chop on each side for 2-4 minutes over high heat.

12. Put on the fresh onion s and fry in the oven for 26 -45 minutes.

13. Pierce with a wooden skewer: If pink meat juice runs out, the chop is still bloody inside.

14. If you do not like it, fry it a few more minutes until the juice that emerges looks bright.

15. Remove the veal chop, wrap in aluminum foil and let rest for 6 minutes.

16. Put the roasting pan on the stove and bring the meat juice to a boil.

17. Deglaze with white wine and bring to a boil.

18. Add the soy cream and cook over medium heat for 4 -4 minutes until creamy.

19. Squeeze 2 teaspoons of juice from the fresh lemon half.

20. Season the sauce with salt, pepper, and fresh lemon juice.

21. Serve with meat.

Sausages Stuffed Mushrooms

INGREDIENTS

- 2 tablespoons cream cheese
- 2 tablespoon of ground flaxseed
- 2 fresh onion
- 2 sausages
- 2 clove of garlic

PREPARATION

a. Remove the intestines and fry the sausage with the pressed garlic.
b. Then place it on the page for later.
c. Then remove the stems of mushrooms and chop them small.

d. Mix the finely chopped champignon stems with the cream cheese and then add the cooled sausage meat.

e. Finally, add the ground flax seeds and fill the mushrooms with the mixture.

f. Place the mushrooms in a large casserole dish and bake at 160 ° C for 26 minutes.

Frittata With Spinach And Grainy Cream Cheese

INGREDIENTS

- 100 g granular cream cheese, 25 % fat i.Tr
- 2 pinch of sea salt
- 2 pinch of black pepper

- 2 tbsp olive oil

- 4 fresh fresh fresh fresh eggs s size M
- 45 g spinach, raw
- 4 tablespoons whipped cream 4 0%
- 6 0 g of Parmesan

PREPARATION

1. Wash the spinach and drain well.

2. Beat the fresh fresh fresh fresh eggs s and stir in a bowl with whipped cream.

3. Add the cream cheese and season with salt and pepper.

4. Stir again.

5. Heat the olive oil in the frying pan and add the fresh fresh fresh eggs mass.

6. Add the spinach leaves and let the fresh fresh fresh eggs mass stagnate over medium heat.

7. Then add freshly grated Parmesan cheese over the fresh fresh fresh eggs mass.

8. Place the frittata in the pan for 16 - 25 minutes in the oven preheated to 180 ° C.

9. Remove the finished frittata from the oven and cut into pieces, sprinkle with freshly squeezed fresh lemon juice and serve.

Cauliflower And Cheese Gressinos

INGREDIENTS

- 4 fresh fresh fresh fresh eggs s
- 2 cc ground oregano

- salt & pepper
- 25 0g Cauliflower
- 6 0g mozzarella cheese

PREPARATION

1. Put the gratin paper into the baking dish.

2. Make sure the cauliflower is cut into a rapier.

153

3. Add rapier to the food processor and beat it until the cauliflower looks like rice.

4. Place the cauliflower in a microwave and place it in a special container with a lid for 2-4 minutes.

5. Remove cauliflower from the microwave and pour into a large bowl.

6. Add 4 fresh fresh fresh fresh eggs s , 40g mozzarella cheese, oregano, garlic, salt, and pepper.

7. Made all the dough and made a dough.

8. Bake only the crust at medium temperature for about 26 minutes or until golden.

9. Once baked, spread the remaining mozzarella cheese and bake for another 6 minutes or until the cheese melts.

10. Served by cutting into bread crumbs.

Hamburger With Brie Cheese And Caramelized Fresh Onion

INGREDIENTS

- 4 mushrooms
- 125 g minced beef

- 2 cc black pepper

- 45 g brie cheese

- 2 cs olive oil
- 6 0 g white fresh onion
- 2 cc salt
- 2 cs butter

PREPARATION

1. Heat olive oil in a large tempura pan and cook the fresh onion s with a pinch of salt for 6 minutes until the caramel color is soft and brownish.

2. Don't be crunchy! Place the fresh onion on a plate, and the flyer is useful for cooking mushrooms.

3. For hamburgers, put meat, salt, and pepper in a large container.

4. Mix by hand and mix well and split into two equal parts.

5. Place on one of brie cheese and fresh onion and place on the other.

6. Cook the hamburger for about 4 minutes on one side and apply the butter to the mushrooms.

7. This takes about 2-4 minutes.

8. Once everything is cooked, add mushrooms and fresh onion s to a hamburger and add the salad.

Cheese Tacos

INGREDIENTS

- tbsp peeled tomatoes, cut into small pieces
- 2 ml tomato puree
- 6 tbsp creme fraiche
- 150 g grated cheese
- 425 g ground beef
- 2 cloves of garlic
- 2 paprika
- tbsp curry spices
- tbsp bell pepper spices

PREPARATION

1. Preheat the oven to 180 °.
2. Take the top board and place the top board on it.
3. Stack 6-8 grated cheese.
4. This cheese is melted in an oven, and a taco shell is made from it.
5. Bake until the cheese is golden in about 10 minutes.
6. Meanwhile, finely chop the fresh onion , garlic, and peppers.
7. When the cheese melts and becomes golden, remove the top board from the oven.
8. Tap the excess fat with a kitchen roll.
9. Next, make your own tacos by bending the cheese into the correct shape.

10. Next, put the minced meat in a frying pan.
11. Stir fresh onion , garlic, and peppers.
12. Fry this for another 6 minutes
13. Add tomato puree and peeled tomatoes.
14. Add salt and pepper to the taste.
15. Stir until all moisture has evaporated.
16. Next, divide the mix into tacos.

17. Finally, add a little creme fresh.

Scrumptious Chicken Bacon Chowder

Ingredients:

- 2 ribs celery, diced
- 2 tsp. garlic powder
- 2 cups chicken stock, divided
- 2 small leek, cleaned, trimmed and sliced
- 6 mushrooms, sliced
- 2 shallot, finely chopped
- 4 cloves garlic, minced
- 4 tbsp. butter, divided
- 2 tsp. dried thyme
- 2 tsp. black pepper
- 2 tsp. sea salt
- 8 oz. cream cheese

- 2 medium sweet fresh onion , thinly sliced
- 2 lb. chicken breasts or thighs
- 2 cup heavy cream

Directions:

1. Turn the cooker on Low.

2. Add the leeks, black pepper, mushrooms, fresh onion s, 2 cup chicken stock, sea salt, 2 tbsp.

3. butter, shallot, celery and garlic into the cooker and stir to combine.

4. Cover and cook for about 45 mins.

5. Heat 2 tbsp. butter in a frying pan over medium heat and pan-sear the chicken breasts until browned on both sides. Set aside.

6. Add the remaining 2 cup of chicken stock to the slow cooker.

7. Add the thyme, heavy cream, cream cheese, and garlic powder into the slow cooker.

8. Carefully stir the ingredients.

Beef And Bacon Meatloaf With Brussels Sprouts And Carrots

Ingredients:

- 2 tsp. salt
- 1 cup cheese, shredded
- 1 tsp. pepper
- 8 oz. sliced bacon
- 2 1/8 cups heavy whipping cream for gravy
- 2 fresh onion , finely chopped
- 2 tbsp. butter
- 26 oz. ground beef
- 2 fresh fresh fresh eggs
- 1 cup heavy whipping cream
- 2 tbsp. dried oregano

Directions:

1. Preheat the oven to 425 °F.

2. In a pan, fry the chopped fresh onion in butter until translucent and tender.

3. In a bowl, mix the ground beef, fresh onion s, fresh fresh fresh eggs   , oregano, salt, heavy whipping cream, cheese, and pepper.

4. Blend the ingredients gently together combining well.

5. Form the combination into a loaf shape and place in a baking dish or loaf pan.

6. Now wrap the loaf with the bacon slices.

7. Bake the bacon-wrapped loaf in the oven for forty-five to fifty minutes.

8. Should the bacon appear to overcook, you can cover the baking dish with some aluminum foil.

9. Pour the juices from the baking plate into a saucepan and add in 2 1/8 cups of heavy whipping cream.

10. Once the gravy boils, set the heat lower and simmer for 16 minutes.

167

CPSIA information can be obtained
at www.ICGtesting.com
Printed in the USA
LVHW081952280223
740558LV00027B/408